Recipes For Homemade Face And Body Products

By

Gene Ashburner

ISBN-13:978-1508814054
ISBN-10:1508814058

Content

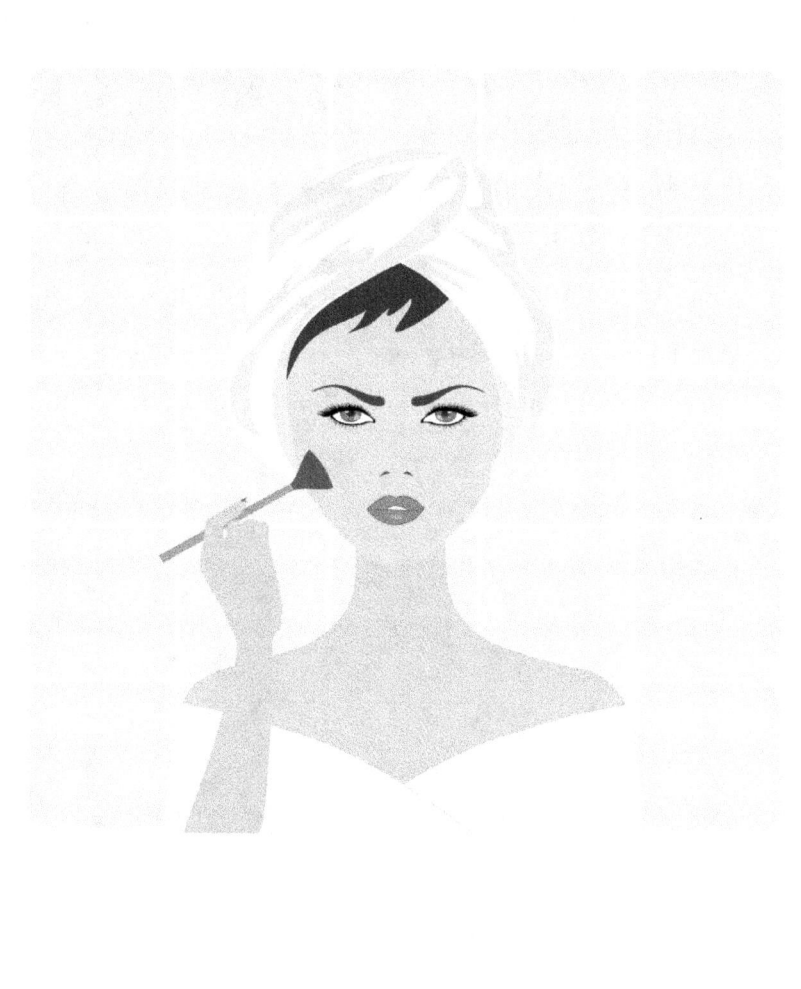

Baby And Children Skin Care

Baby Wipes Recipe 1

Ingredients

62,5 ml aloe vera juice

4 drops lavender oil

1/2 roll paper towels (cut lengthwise)

62,5 ml water

2 drops tea tree oil

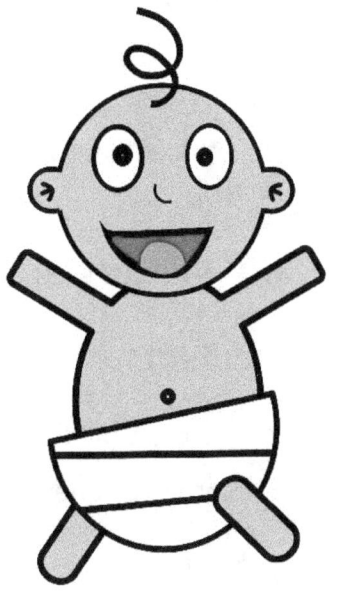

Method

Combine all the ingredients together.

Store the wipes in a plastic container.

Baby Wipes Recipe 2

Ingredients

1 roll strong paper towel

500 ml water

125 ml almond oil

125 ml organic baby wash

Method

Cut the paper towel in half.

Take out the cardboard inner roll.

Combine the water, almond oil and baby wash together.

Place one half of the roll into a container and pour over ½ of the solution.

Store the "wipes" in the container.

Baby Wiping Solution

Ingredients

250 ml chamomile tea

5 ml organic honey

Method

Combine all the ingredients together.

Mix well.

Use to wipe down the baby.

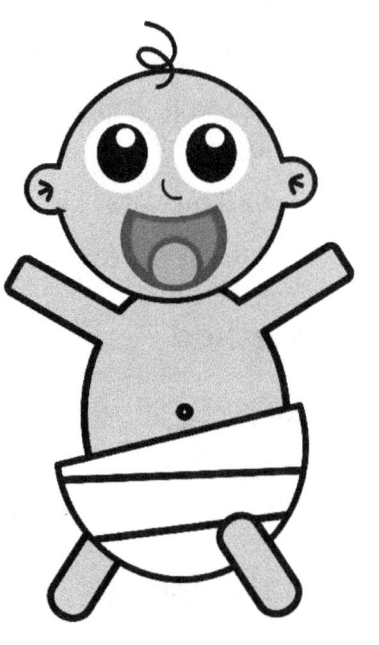

Cradle Cap Care

Ingredients

Sweet almond oil

Method

Wipe the affected area with sweet almond oil.

Leave on for 10 minutes.

Wash baby's scalp with an organic baby wash or shampoo.

Do not leave the oil on the scalp as this will cause further dryness.

Oatmeal Bath

When baby's skin gets very itchy from eczema, an oatmeal bath can be very soothing and help skin heal.

Ingredients

500 ml oats (ground to a powder)

Method

Add the oatmeal powder to a running bath of warm water.

Mix well.

Let the baby soak in the oatmeal bath for 15 minutes.

Rinse with clean water and dab the skin dry with a soft towel.

When baby's eczema breakouts are bad, it is safe to sooth them with an oatmeal bath twice daily.

Skin Wash

This natural skin wash is very gentle for your baby and helps with itching caused by eczema.

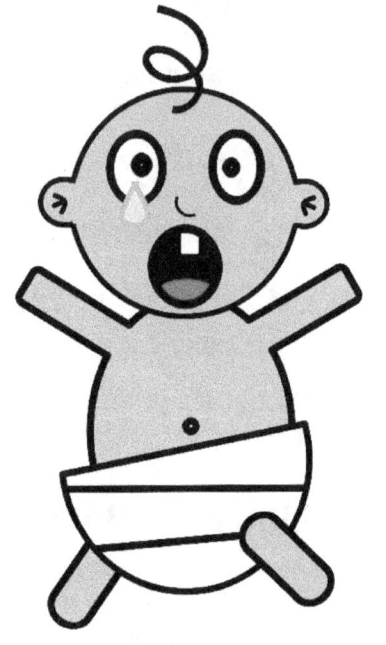

Ingredients

5 ml comfrey root

5 ml white oak bark

5 ml slippery elm bark

500 ml water

Method

Combine comfrey root, white oak bark, slippery elm bark and water together in a saucepan.

Mix well.

Bring to a boil over a medium heat.

Simmer for 30 minutes.

Allow the mixture to cool.

Strain out the solids.

Use the liquid like any face wash.

Soap Crayons for Kid's Bath

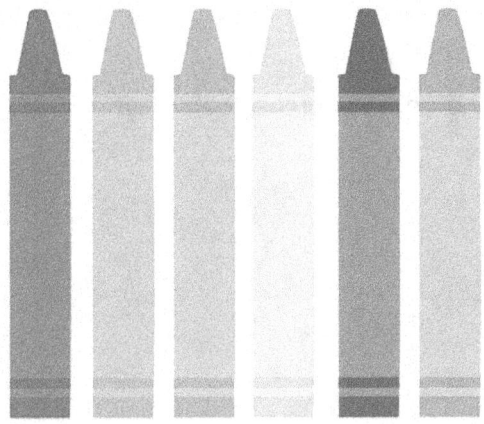

Ingredients

250 ml soap flakes

62,5 ml boiling water

Food coloring (different colors)

Ice cube tray

Method

Combine the water and soap flakes together.

Stir constantly, it will be thick and hard to stir.

Divide the soap into different bowls.

Color each bowl with the food coloring and stir until it has the consistency of a thick paste.

Press spoonfuls of the soap mixture into the ice cube trays.

Microwave the soap on low for 15 minutes.

Leave the soap to dry at room temperature for several days.

Unmold the soap crayons.

Leave for 1 day before using the soap crayons.

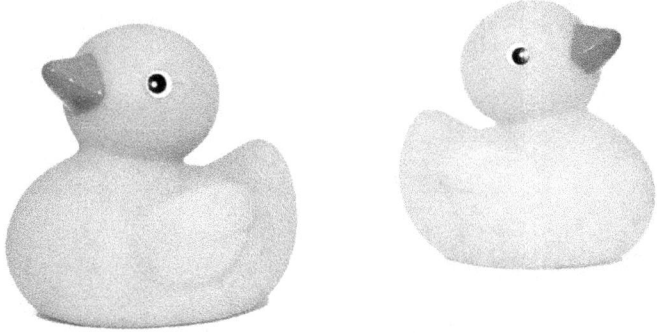

Bath Products

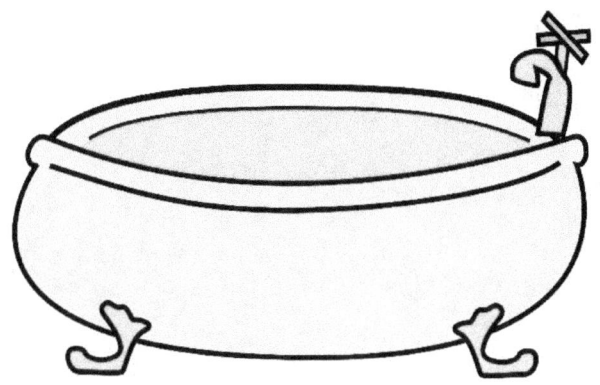

Bath Salts

Ingredients

1000 ml Epsom salt

500 ml sea salt

1 1/2 ml glycerin

2 to 3 drops food coloring

5 to 6 drops essential oil fragrance (vanilla, peppermint, strawberry)

Method

Combine all ingredients together.

Mix well.

Spread the mixture out to dry.

Spoon the bath salts into jars.

Bubble Bath

Ingredients

1 quart distilled water (warm)

1 bar castile soap (grated – see below)

2 oz liquid glycerine (helps to create bubbles)

4 drops essential oil of choice (see below)

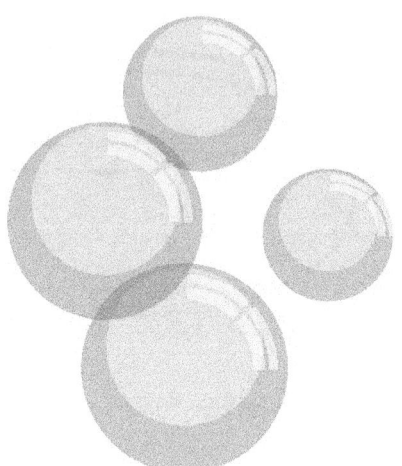

Soothing

♦ Lavender, rosewood, sandalwood, chamomile and myrrh.

Energizing and rejuvenating

♦ Eucalyptus, spearmint, peppermint, and lemon oil.

Softening the skin

♦ Almond and coconut oil.

Castile Soap

♦ This type of soap was originally made from olive oil although other types of oils can also be used, such as: coconut, almond, hemp, and jojoba.

Method

Combine the water and soap together.

Mix until all the soap has dissolved.

Add the glycerin and essential oil.

Mix gently.

Bubble Bath For The Winter Months

Here is a bubble bath recipe to soak in when you're sick. Eucalyptus can help your body fight cold symptoms and reduce congestion.

Ingredients

6 drops eucalyptus oil

3 drops spearmint oil

3 drops peppermint oil

1 quart distilled water (heated)

1 bar castile soap (grated – see below)

4 oz liquid glycerine

Castile Soap

This type of soap was originally made from olive oil although other types of oils can also be used, such as: coconut, almond, hemp, and jojoba.

Method

Combine the water and soap together.

Mix until the soap has dissolved.

Add the remaining ingredients.

Mix gently.

Store the mixture in a bottle.

Citronella Soap

Ingredients

250 ml castile soap (grated – see below)

125 ml water (boiling)

10 drops citronella essential oil

5 drops eucalyptus essential oil

12,5 ml pennyroyal leaves (dried and crushed)

Castile Soap

This type of soap was originally made from olive oil although other types of oils can also be used, such as: coconut, almond, hemp, and jojoba.

Method

Combine the soap and water together.

Mix until the soap has dissolved.

Add the remaining ingredients.

Whip the soap with an electric beater until the mixture has doubled in volume.

Spoon the soap into the prepared molds.

The beating action cools the mixture so work quickly.

Elbows

Darkened Elbow Remedy 1

Ingredients

25 ml lemon juice

25 ml cream

Method

Combine the lemon juice and cream together.

Apply the mixture onto the elbows.

Leave for 30 minutes.

Rinse off with tepid water.

Darkened Elbow Remedy 2

Ingredients

25 ml cucumber juice

25 ml lemon juice

Method

Combine the ingredients together.

Apply the mixture onto the elbows.

Leave for 15 minutes.

Rinse off with tepid water.

Facial Cleansers And Masks

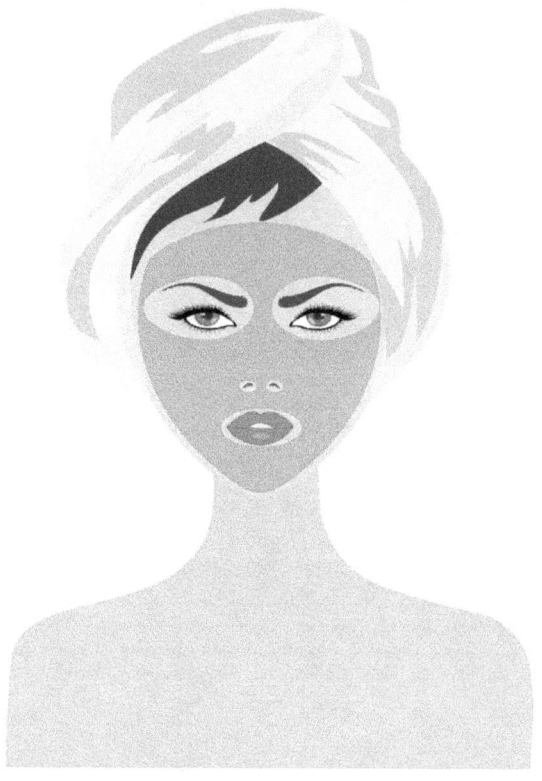

Making one's own natural facial cleanser ensures that the daily build–up of dirt is gently washed away without stripping away the skin's essential natural attributes. In order to maximize the benefits of using a natural facial cleanser, apply the homemade recipe to warm moist skin. Use a circular motion to gently massage the skin with the cleanser, then rinse well. This face wash strategy will ensure a deep cleansing of clogging dirt from the pores which will then leave the skin clean, soft and supple.

Acne Mask

Ingredients

1 egg white (beaten stiff)

1 drop lemon juice – oily skin

5 ml organic honey – dry skin

Method

Add either the lemon juice or the honey to the egg white.

Apply it over your face.

Leave for 20 minutes.

Rinse off with water.

Rinse your face first with warm water and then with cold water after you finish removing the mask.

Apply the facial mask once a week.

Acne Remedy 1

Ingredients

Distilled white vinegar

Method

Apply the vinegar to the face and affected acne areas.

Leave for 5 to 10 minutes.

Rinse off with cool water.

Acne Remedy 2

Ingredients

20 ml organic honey

1 apple (peeled, cored and grated)

Method

Combine the honey and apple together.

Apply the paste to your face.

Leave for 10 minutes.

Rinse the face with warm water.

Repeat the procedure twice a week.

Apple Mask

Use For: normal skin

Ingredients

1 apple (peeled, cored and quartered)

25 ml honey

Method

Blend the apple and honey in a blender until smooth.

Remove the mixture from the blender.

Refrigerate for 10 minutes.

Apply the mixture to your face using a patting motion and be sure to pat until the honey becomes tacky.

Leave it on for 30 minutes.

Rinse with warm water.

Aspirin Mask

Use For: cleaning pores from deep inside and keeping skin blemish-free

Indications

All skin types, especially normal to oily and combination skin, acne-prone and clogged skin

Ingredients

3 to 5 plain aspirin (crushed)

Distilled water

Method

Combine the aspirin powder with the water until creamy.

Apply on clean dry skin (focus on T-zone and sides of the nose).

Keep it on until completely dry.

Take a small cotton pad, wet it lightly and begin scrubbing the areas covered with the mask, making small circles.

Rinse off with plenty of water.

Variations

Add yoghurt for an astringent effect

Add aloe vera

Add honey

Banana Yogurt Mask

Use For: skin treatment

Ingredients

½ ripe banana (peeled and mashed)

12,5 ml organic honey

12,5 ml wheat germ

12,5 ml plain yogurt

Method

Combine all the ingredients together.

Mix well.

Apply to your face.

Leave for 15 minutes.

Rinse off with tepid water.

Cucumber Mask

Use For: skin care moisturizer

Ingredients

10 ml uncooked oatmeal

12,5 ml extra-virgin olive oil

¼ cucumber (pureed)

12,5 ml organic honey

Method

Combine all the ingredients together to form a thick paste.

Apply the mask to your face.

Leave for 15 minutes.

Rinse with tepid water.

Deep Cleansing Mask

Ingredients

1/2 cucumber (peeled and pureed)

12,5 ml plain yogurt

Method

Combine all the ingredients together.

Apply to the face.

Leave for 20 minutes.

Rinse off with warm water.

Use once or twice a week to remove dead skin cells and refresh your skin.

Egg White Mask

Use For: whitening skin care treatment

Ingredients

> 12,5 ml organic honey
>
> 1 egg white (slightly beaten)
>
> 25 ml unflavored gelatine

Method

Combine the gelatin and honey together.

Add the egg white.

Mix well.

Apply the mask on your face.

Leave for 15 minutes.

Rinse with tepid water.

Peach Mask

Use For: tightening mask

Ingredients

1 ripened peach (peeled and pitted)

1 egg white

Method

Blend the peach and egg white together in a blender until smooth.

Remove from blender.

Pat the mixture onto your face.

Leave for 30 minutes.

Rinse with cold water.

Oatmeal Mask

Use For: very oily skin, using an oatmeal mask can bring about substantive results

Ingredients

Oatmeal

Water

Method

Combine the water and oatmeal to form a paste.

Apply the paste to your face.

Leave for 20 minutes.

Rinse the paste off with cold water.

Apply this mask twice a day.

Strawberry Mask

Use For: normal skin

Ingredients

125 ml strawberries (very ripe)

125 ml cornstarch

Method

Blend the strawberries and cornstarch together in a blender until smooth.

Remove from the blender.

Apply the mixture to your face and be careful to avoid the area around your eyes.

Leave for 30 minutes.

Rinse it off with cool water.

Tomato Mask

Use For: blemished skin

Ingredients

1 ripe tomato (skinned and chopped)

12,5 ml lemon juice

25 ml rolled oats

Method

Blend the tomato, lemon juice and rolled oats together in a blender until all combined (do not mix for too long, as it will not stick to your face).

If it gets too thin add more rolled oats.

Apply the mixture to your face.

Leave for 10 minutes.

Scrub it off using a warm, wet cloth.

Exfoliator

Lemon or any citric fruit works great as a natural exfoliate, removing dead skin cells that may clog the pours.

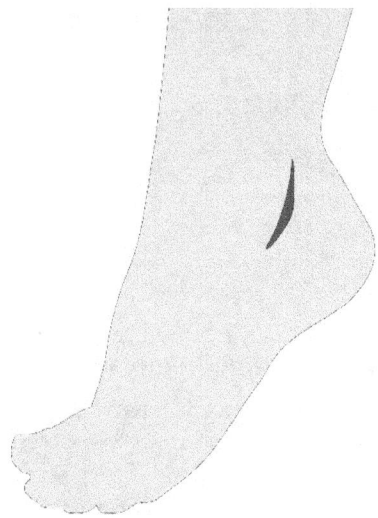

Ingredients

Juice of 1 lemon

Method

Apply the lemon juice to the face.

Leave for 10 minutes.

Rinse with cool water.

Exfoliator – Sugar

Ingredients

Olive oil

Sugar

Method

After cleaning face and rinsing completely cover face with olive oil.

Apply granulated sugar over the oil.

Gently roll the sugar mixture across the skin.

Use small circular motions.

After sugar dissolves use warm water and a good cleanser to wash the solution away. Rinse at least a dozen of times to thoroughly remove the alkaline residue.

Facial Cleanser For Normal To Oily Skin

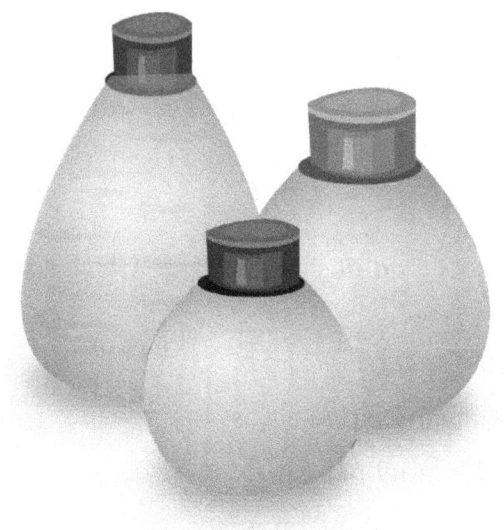

Ingredients

25 ml cornstarch

25 ml glycerin

125 ml distilled water

Method

Combine all the ingredients together until smooth.

Pour the mixture into a jar.

Place the jar inside a double-boiler.

Bring the water in the outer pot to boiling point.

Heat the mixture until it is clear and has thickened.

Remove from the heat and allow the mixture to cool.

The cleanser can be kept for 7 to 10 days.

Facial Scrub For Blackheads

Ingredients

25 ml baking soda

25 ml water

Method

Combine the ingredients together to form a paste.

Gently scrub the blackheads for 2 to 3 minutes.

Rinse off with tepid water.

Use once or twice a week.

Facial Scrub For Oily Skin

Ingredients

25 ml sea salt

25 ml lemon juice

Method

Combine the ingredients together to form a paste.

Gently scrub the face for 1 to 2 minutes.

Rinse off with tepid water.

Use once a week to remove dead skin cells.

Green Tea Skin Toner

Ingredients

1 green tea teabag

125 ml boiling water

4 drops tea tree oil

Method

Steep the teabag in the boiling water for 2 to 3 minutes.

Remove the tea bag.

Allow the water cool.

Add the tea tree oil.

Pour the cooled water into a bottle.

Use with cotton pads like you would regular toner.

Pimple Remedies

Remedy 1

♦ Apply a paste of fresh fenugreek leaves over the face.

♦ Leave for 15 minutes.

♦ Rinse with warm water.

♦ This will prevent pimples, blackheads, and wrinkles.

Remedy 2

♦ Apply raw papaya juice, including the skin and seeds onto swelling pimples.

♦ Leave for 15 minutes.

♦ Rinse with warm water.

♦ This will prevent pimples.

Remedy 3

♦ Apply fresh lime juice mixed with a glass of boiled milk as a face wash for pimples.

Remedy 4

♦ Mix lime juice and rose water in equal portions.

♦ Apply on affected area.

♦ Leave for 30 minutes.

♦ Rinse off with lukewarm water.

Remedy 5

♦ Apply ripe tomatoes pulp on pimples.

♦ Leave for 1 hour.

♦ Rinse off with tepid water.

Remedy 6

♦ Grind nutmeg with un-boiled milk and apply on affected area.

♦ Pimples should disappear without leaving a mark.

Remedy 7

♦ Make a paste by mixing 37,5 ml honey and 5 ml cinnamon together.

♦ Apply this paste on the pimples before sleeping.

♦ Wash it off the next morning with warm water.

♦ Repeat for two weeks, pimples will disappear forever.

Remedy 8

♦ Apply a mixture of 1 teaspoon lemon juice and 1 teaspoon cinnamon powder.

Remedy 9

♦ Grind orange zest and water together to form a paste.

♦ Apply on and around pimples.

Remedy 10

♦   Rub fresh garlic on and around pimples.

♦   Pimples will disappear without a mark with regular applications.

Remedy 11

♦   Combine 12,5 ml groundnut oil and 12,5 ml limejuice together.

♦   Rub onto your face.

♦   This will prevent formation of blackheads and pimples.

Remedy 12

♦   Apply fresh mint juice over the face every night for the treatment of pimples, insect stings, eczema, scabies and other skin infections.

Skin Toner

Use For: skin tightening and closing pores

Ingredients

5 drops grapefruit seed extract

62,5 ml witch hazel

125 ml apple cider vinegar

Method

Combine the grapefruit seed extract, witch hazel and apple cider vinegar together.

Mix well.

Use this as a toner after you have washed your face.

Hair

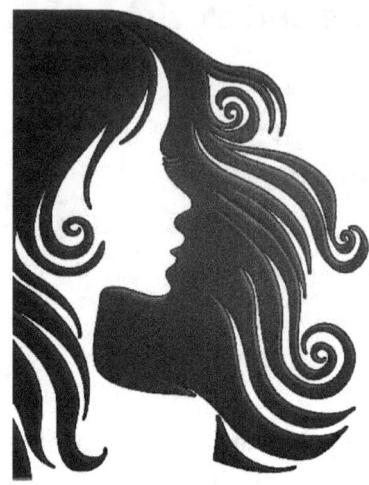

Scalp Hair Rinse

Use For: This helps control dandruff

Ingredients

    500 ml apple cider vinegar (heated to boiling point)

    62, 5ml sage, rosemary and thyme (dried and crushed)

Method

Combine the boiling apple cider vinegar and the herbs.

Cover and leave for 10 minutes.

Strain the mixture.

Pour the liquid into a bottle.

Feet

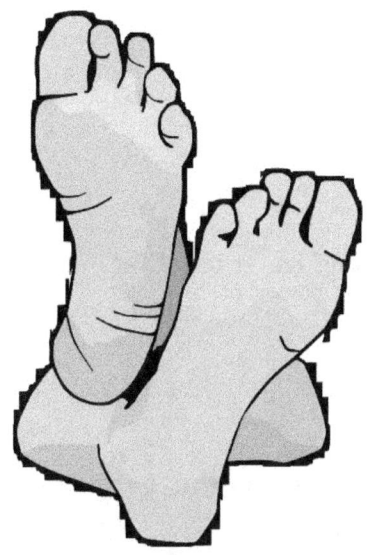

Herbal Footbath

Ingredients

37,5 ml herbal mix (see below)

375 ml water

Herbal Mix

♦ Dandelion root

♦ Yellow dock root

♦ Saraparilla root

- Echinacea
- Licorice
- Kelp
- Chaparral
- Fresh Garlic

Method

Combine the herbal mix and water together in a saucepan.

Bring the mixture to the boil.

Remove from the heat.

Leave for 30 minutes.

The longer the tea sits the stronger the tea and its effects.

Prepare your foot spa with water.

Strain the tea to remove the leaves and roots.

Pour the tea into the foot spa.

Place your feet the water for 15 to 30 minutes.

Hands

Soft Hands

Use For: maintain them in a good condition

Ingredients

Almond oil

Method

Massage hands with almond oil.

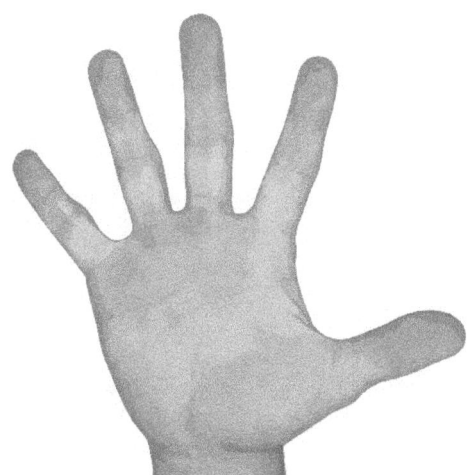

Stained Hands

Ingredients

Lemon juice

Method

Rub a little lemon juice onto the stain after washing your hands but before drying them.

Lips

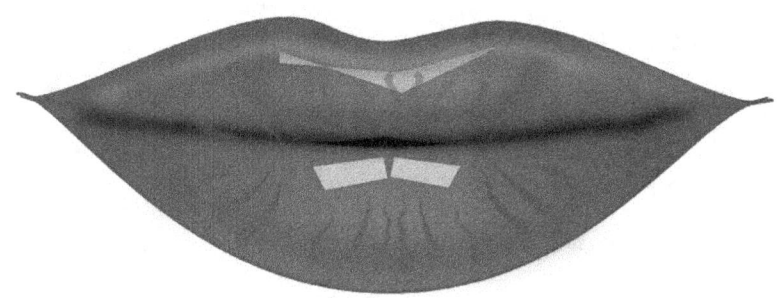

Lip Balm And Lip Gloss

Ingredients

62,5 ml nut oil

1/4 oz beeswax

5 ml honey

5 drops essential oil (never use extracts found in cooking sections as they contain alcohol – use Comfrey, Rosemary, Tea Tree or Camphor Oils)

Few drops beetroot juice

Method

Heat the nut oil and beeswax in a double boiler until the beeswax has melted.

Remove from the heat.

Whip the mixture with an electric beater until creamy.

Add the honey, essential oil and beetroot juice.

Whip the mixture again.

Store the lip gloss / balm in small glass jars.

If the balm is too hard (waxy) add more oil to your mixture.

If the balm is too soft add more wax.

Don't use food colouring as it may contain alcohol base.

Basic Lip Gloss

Ingredients

1 ½ ml paraffin wax (grated)

Ziploc bag

5 ml coconut oil

5 ml petroleum jelly

1 candy melt

0.63 ml oil-based candy flavouring

Grater

Method

Place the wax into the plastic bag.

Add the coconut oil, petroleum jelly and candy melt.

Add the candy flavouring.

Seal the plastic bag and place it into a bowl of hot tap water to melt the ingredients.

When all the ingredients are melted remove the bag from the water.

Mix the ingredients bag by shaking it gently.

Clip off a tiny corner of the bag and squeeze the lip gloss into a clean container.

Leave for 1 hour.

Use a cotton swab to apply the lip-gloss to your lips.

Sunburn Treatments

Tea Tree Oil Remedy 1

Ingredients

25 ml tea tree oil

250 ml olive oil or coconut oil

Method

Combine the ingredients together.

Mix well.

Spread freely over the sunburned area.

It is soothing and pain-relieving and also reduces blistering and peeling.

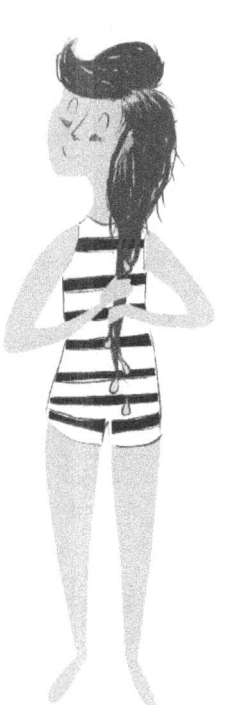

Tea Tree Oil Remedy 2

Ingredients

5 drops tea tree oil

11 drops lavender oil

3 oz distilled water (cold)

Method

Combine the tea tree, lavender oil and water together.

Pour the mixture into a bottle with a spray atomizer.

Spray the mist onto the sunburned areas whenever cooling relief is needed.

Cool Milk Compresses

The fat and lactic acids in milk are known to have soothing qualities for sunburned skin

Ingredients

Whole milk (cold)

Cotton gauze

Method

Soak the cotton gauze in the milk.

Dab carefully onto the burned skin.

Do this for 20 minutes.

Rinse off with cool water.

Cool Sugarless Tea As Sunburn Remedy

The tannin in tea is the active ingredient here, which helps to soothe and relieve some of the discomfort of sunburned skin.

Ingredients

Tea bags

Water

Method

Brew a big pot of tea.

Cool the tea completely.

Sponge the cool tea on the affected areas.

Use the cool used teabags for the sensitive areas around the eyes – simply place the teabags over your eyes if they feel hot and tired.

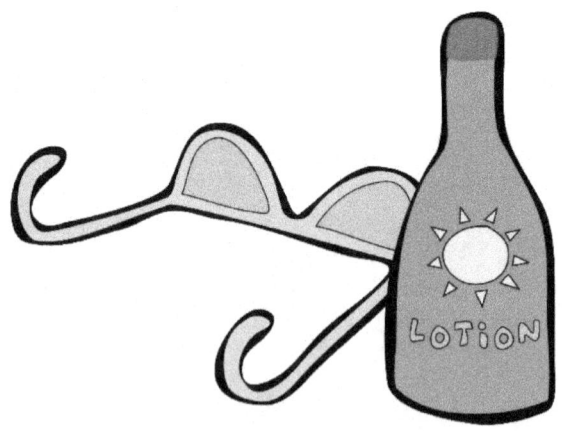

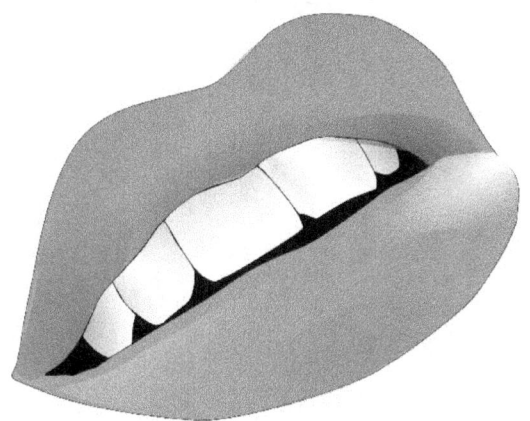

Teeth Whitening Paste

Ingredients

15 ml hydrogen peroxide

10 ml baking soda

Method

Combine the hydrogen peroxide and baking soda together.

Mix well.

Use a toothbrush and leave the mixture on your teeth for at a 2 or 3 minutes.

You should avoid swallowing the paste.

If you do swallow some whitening paste drink lots of water.